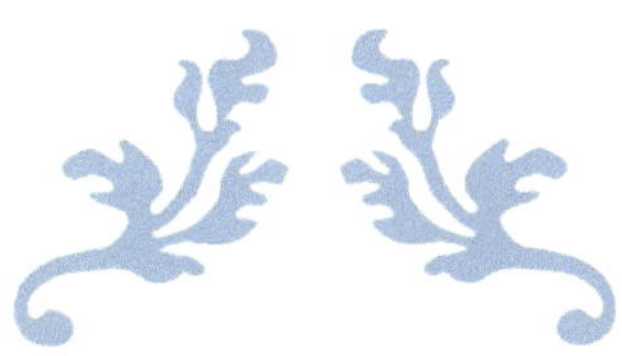

EXERCISES TO ENJOY YOUR GOLDEN YEARS

Written by Barbara Miller

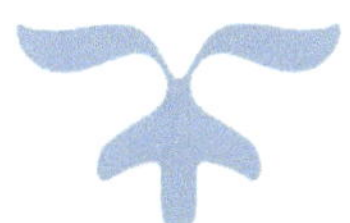

BARBARA MILLER SELF-PUBLISHING

Exercises

To Enjoy

Your Golden Years

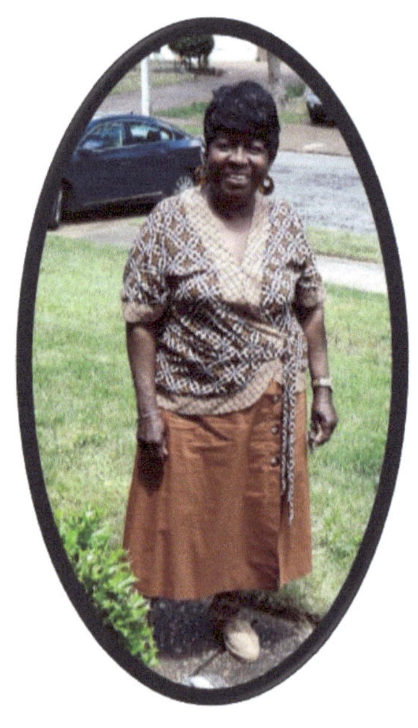

Author Barbara Miller

Introduction

Thanks for joining our Special Group.

 I am 76 years old.

One morning I woke up and it felt like
I had been glued to that one spot where I was lying.

I started to move my left leg, but it hurt something awful.
Even though my left leg was hurting, I moved my left leg slowly
away from My right leg.

I Kept Exercising Lying in My Bed.

I will demonstrate how "We Can Enjoy Our Golden Years".
This book was design to help (us) Seniors move and stay on a
healthier path for life.

While there are plenty of Media with Exercise Activities,
this Book was written especially for Seniors.

This Book is designed to demonstrate Exercises that you can do
no matter WHERE You are or How Old You Are.

 Excising raises your heart rate and increase the circulation of
your blood Flow as it did years ago but at a more moderate rate.

This book guides you step by step by demonstrating each exercise.

 YOU will get a chance to exercise in your bed, standing, or sitting in a chair.
You do not need to put on exercise clothing.

Exercise to enjoy your golden years

Holy Scriptures

Deuteronomy 6:3 (KJV)
3 Hear therefore, O Israel, and observe to do it; that it may be well with thee, and that ye may increase mightily, as the LORD God of thy fathers hath promised thee, in the land that flowed with milk and honey.

Deuteronomy 6:7 (KJV)
7 And thou shalt teach them diligently unto thy children, and shalt talk of them when thou sittest in thine house, and when thou walkest by the way, and when thou liest down, and when thou risest up.

Deuteronomy 6:8 (KJV)
8 And thou shalt bind them for a sign upon thine hand, and they shall be as frontlets between thine eyes.

Why?

Exercise allow our blood to circulate through our body in an extremely healthy manner.

Exercises helps our heart rate to increase to help our hearts to perform at optimum levels.

As mature seniors we should eat food that high in fiber, proteins, and nutrients.

Fiber, nutrients, and exercises work together to nourish our body systems, and to clean out impurities from our systems.

Disclaimer, before you take vitamins, and supplements ask your doctor first, so that the vitamins do not conflict with medicines that you may be taking.

The human body needs water daily to keep the body hydrated, and helps keep the muscles supple, strong, and vibrant.

All scriptures in this book have been extracted from the Holy Bible (Nelson KJV Concordance Copyright 1968 by World Publishing)

This book is designed for mature adults to continue to exercise and to enjoy their "Golden Years!"

Pictures of the equipment for the water exercises were retrieved from the *Independent Living Centers Australia* Website.

Feel to wear whatever you feel comfortable in during the exercises

Acknowledgements

I would like to thank Henry Epps for helping me to achieve one of my life's goal and vision for publishing a book.

I would like to thank all of my friends and family members for listening to me and supporting me through all of my endeavors.

A special thanks to my beautiful children Kenneth C. Miller, Tempra J. Campanella, Booker J. Miller, and Amelia Y. Hunter. They are also my board of directors.

Barbara Miller Self-Publising

Exercises for Mature Adults

Table of Contents

Section 1

Sitting

Leg exercises

Section 1- Sitting Leg Exercises

Chair Exercise

Left Leg Movement to the Left

Directions

Sit in a chair with firm buttock support.

Put both feet firmly flat on the floor.

1. Take a moment to relax in the correct sitting posture.

2. Move the left foot slowly to your left a short distance .

3. Rest a second and move the left foot back to the right to the previous position.

Repeat this exercise several times as you desire and rest between each exercise.

Note: This activity flexes the muscles in your left hip, leg, and foot. This activity also helps in the circulation of your blood.

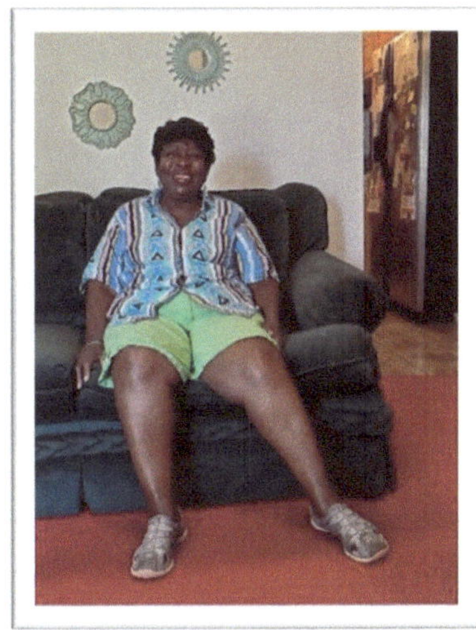

Chair Exercise

Right   Leg Movement to the Right

Directions

Sit in a chair with firm buttock support.

Put both feet firmly flat on the floor.

1. Take a moment to relax in the correct sitting posture.

2. Move the right foot slowly to your right a short distance .

3. Rest a second and move the right foot back to the left to the previous position.

Repeat this exercise several times as you desire and rest between each exercise.

Note: This activity flexes the muscles in your right hip, leg, and foot. This activity also helps in the circulation of your blood.

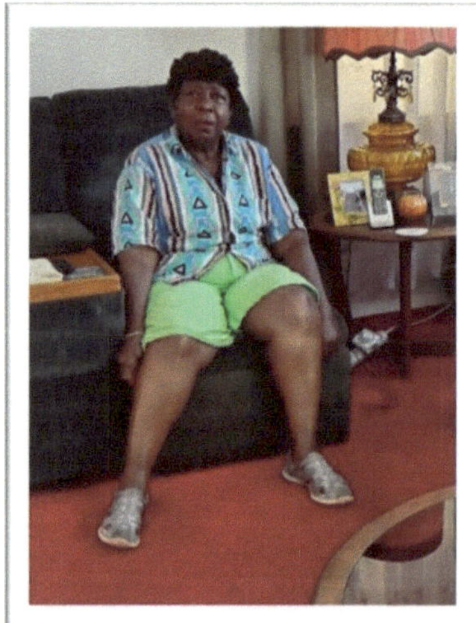

Right leg exercise

Alternate leg Exercises

Directions

Sit in the chair with back straight and bottom firm

Put both feet firmly flat on the floor

Take a moment to relax in the correct sitting position

Move the left foot out to the left about twelve inches

After five seconds return your left foot back to the starting position

Move right foot out to the right about twelve inches and after five seconds move your right back to the starting position

Repeat this exercise and alternate moving the left foot out twelve inches and return to starting position and then move right foot out to twelve inches

Continue this process at least ten repetitions

Seated alternating leg exercise

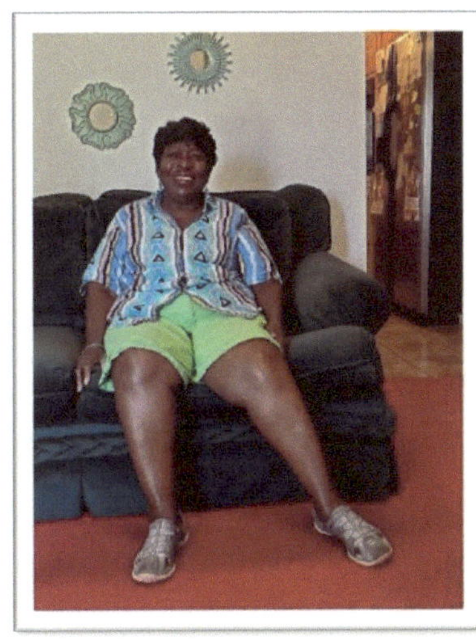
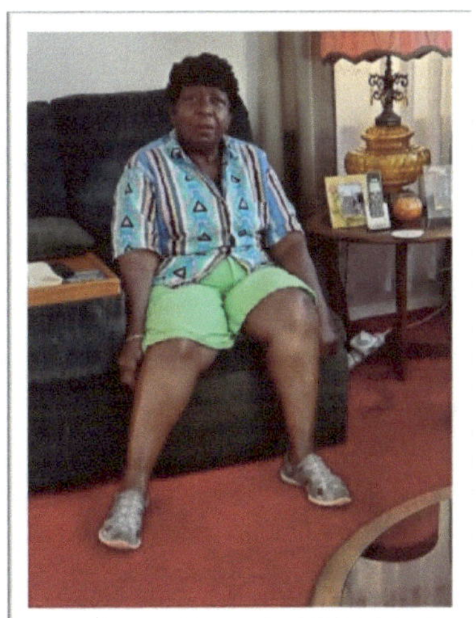

Chair Exercises
Knee lift exercise

Directions
Sit in a chair with back straight and firm for buttock support

Put both feet firmly flat on the floor

Take a moment to relax in the correct sitting posture

Raise left knee about six to eight inches off of the ground

Hold the knee in these position for about five seconds

Lower knee to the original position keeping feet flat on the ground

Repeat this exercise for five repetitions

Right knee lift exercises

Sit in a chair with back straight and firm for buttock support

Put both feet firmly flat on the floor

Take a moment to relax in the correct sitting posture

Raise right knee about six to eight inches off of the ground

Hold the knee in these position for about five seconds

Lower knee to the original position keeping feet flat on the ground

Repeat this exercise for five repetitions

14

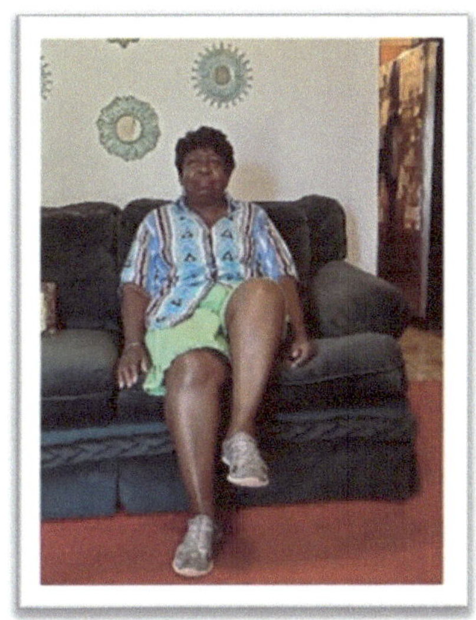
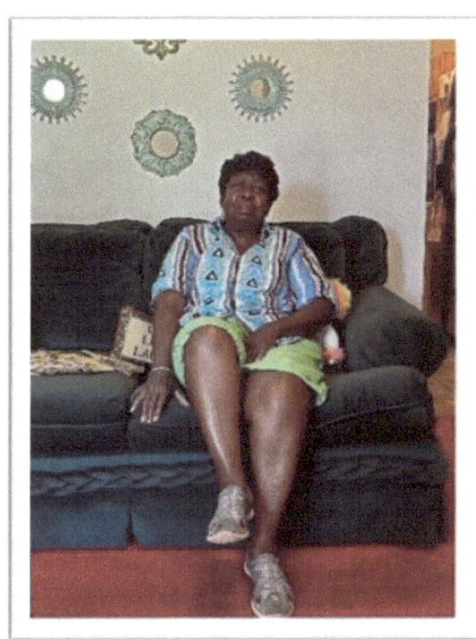

Alternate Knee Exercises

Directions

Sit in the chair with back straight and bottom firm

Put both feet firmly flat on the floor

Take a moment to relax in the correct sitting position

Move the left foot out to the left about twelve inches

After five seconds return your foot back to the starting position

Move right foot out to the right about twelve inches and after five seconds return to starting position

Repeat the first exercise ad alternate moving the left foot out twelve inches and return to starting position and then move right foot out to twelve inches

Continue this process at least ten repetitions

Knee lift exercises

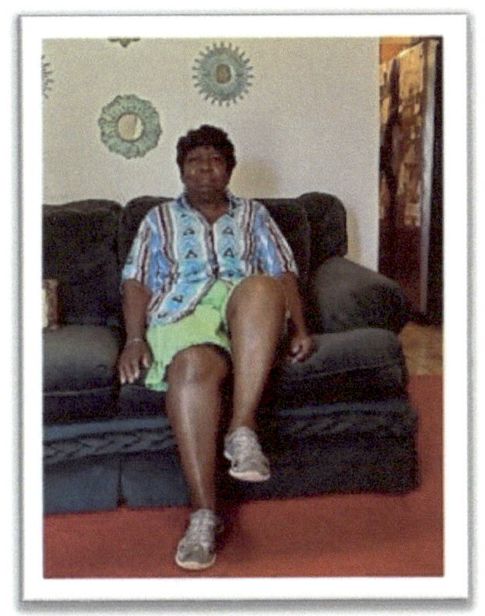
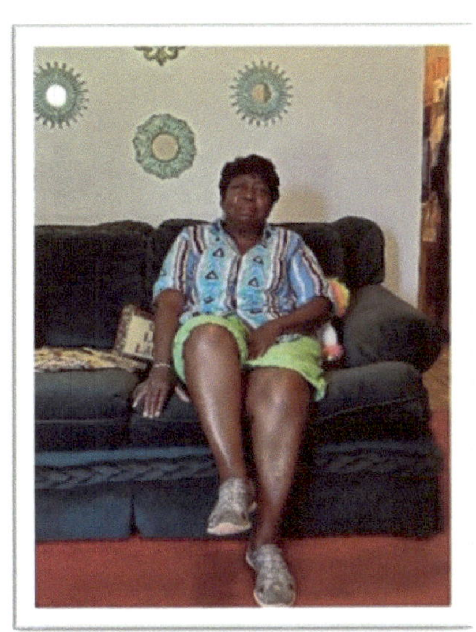

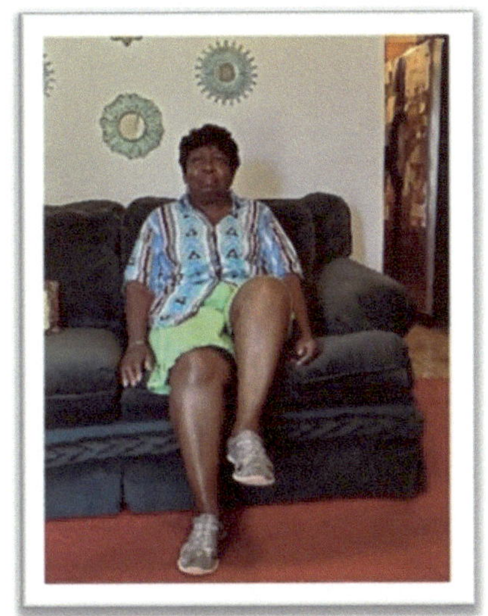
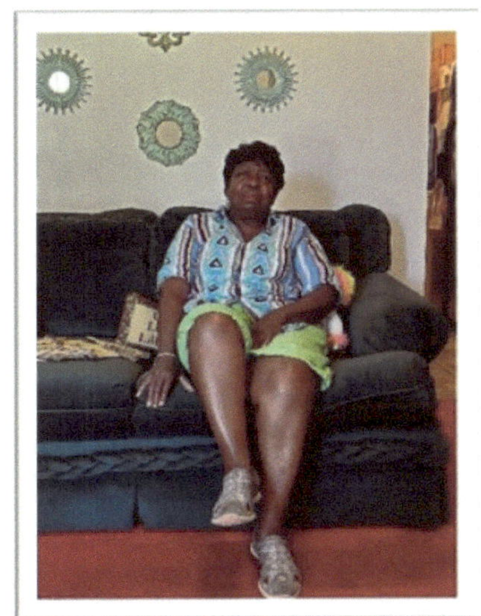

17

Section Two

Lying Down

Exercises

Section 2 -Lying down in your bed exercises

Directions: your bed should have firm support for your whole body.

Stretch out your legs with your toes pointed to the foot of the bed

Arms should be straight along the side of your body

Toes should pointed out towards the foot of your bed

See example

Lying Down leg exercises

Directions:
Slowly move your left leg slowly farther to the left.
Hold in place for a few seconds.
Slowly move your left leg back to the previous.

Rest   Relax   repeat

Slowly move your left leg slowly farther to the left.
Hold in place for a few seconds.
Slowly move your left leg back to the previous.
Rest   Relax   Switch

Slowly move your right leg slowly farther to the right.
Hold in place for a few seconds.
Slowly move your right leg back to the previous.

Rest   Relax   repeat

Slowly move your right leg slowly farther to the right.
Hold in place for a few seconds.
Slowly move your right leg back to the previous.

Alternating Leg Movement Lying Down

Slowly move your left leg slowly farther to the left.
Hold in place for a few seconds.
Slowly move your left leg back to the previous.

Rest   Relax   Switch

Slowly move your right leg slowly farther to the right.
Hold in place for a few seconds.
Slowly move your right leg back to the previous.

Rest   Relax   Switch

Left leg exercise

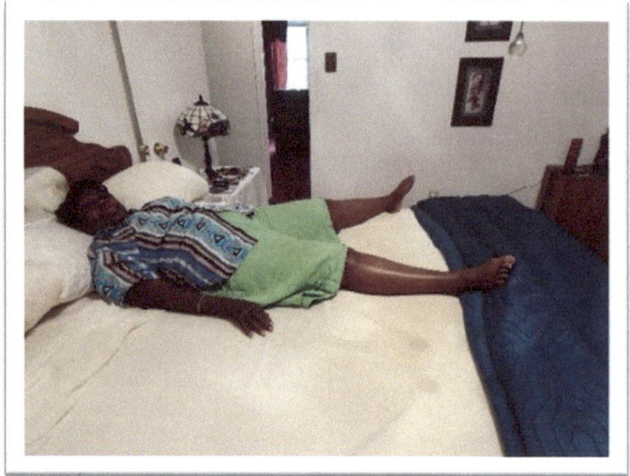

Right Leg Exercise

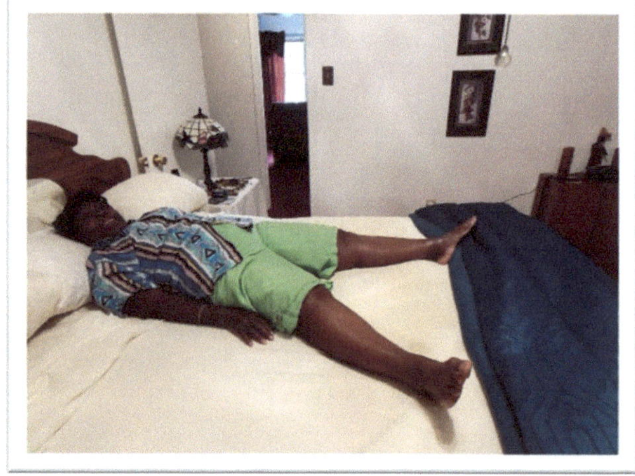

Upper body Lying down exercise

Directions

This exercise is for the upper body

Lay down on your bed

Relax and be comfortable

Stretch out your right arm above your head as far as you can without straining yourself

Hold for five seconds and then return to the starting position

Repeat this exercise for ten repetitions and two sets

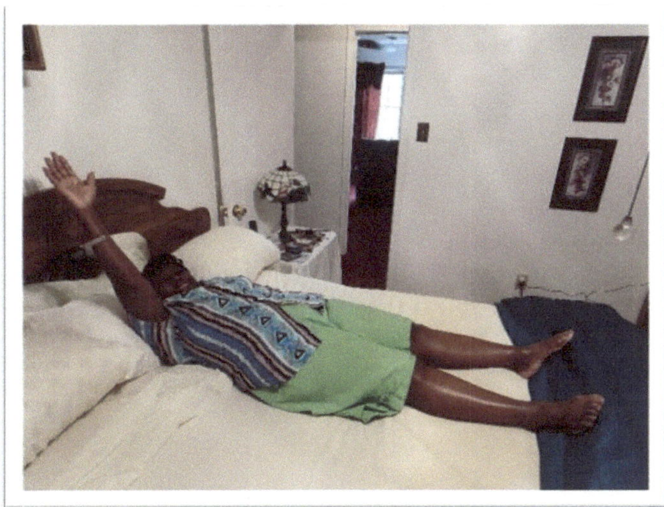

Upper body exercise lying down arm raise

Upper body Lying down exercise

Directions

This exercise is for the upper body

Lay down on your bed

Relax and be comfortable

Stretch out your left arm above your head as far as you can without straining yourself

Hold for five seconds and then return to the starting position

Repeat this exercise for ten repetitions and two sets

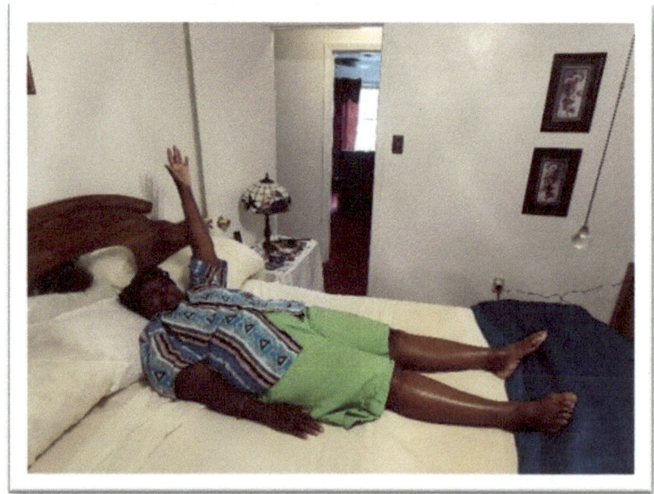

Left Arm raise exercise

Alternating left and right arm exercise

Directions

Begin by laying on your bed and get comfortable

The starting position while laying down with your arms along the side of your body palms facing downward

Raise your right hand over your head with fingers extended and hold for five seconds

Lower your hand back to your side

Alternate and raise your left hand above your head and hold for five seconds

Lower your left hand back to your side and repeat exercise one by raising your right hand and holding for five seconds

Repeat this exercise for 10 repetitions and 2 sets

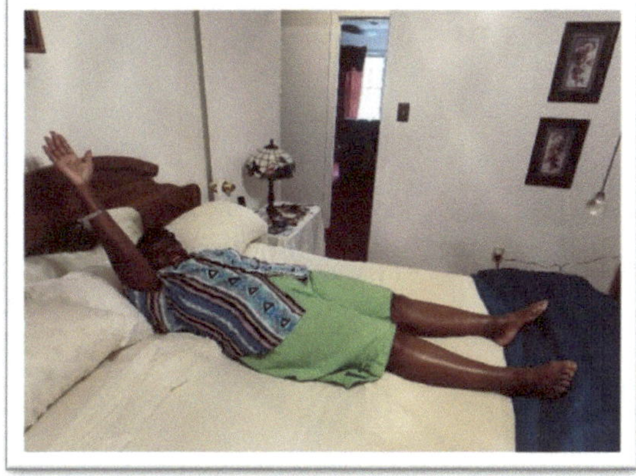
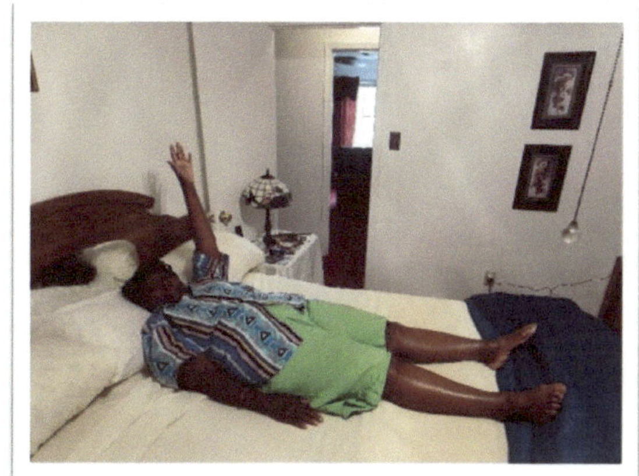

Section three

Walk-in-Bathtub

Exercise

Section 3- Exercises for sitting in heated Walk-in-Tub

Example of a Walk-in-Tub

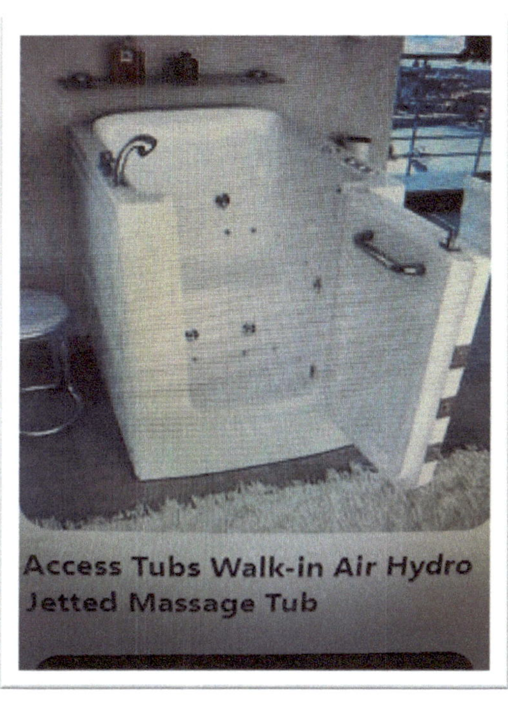

Directions

Take a comfortable seat in your walk-in-Tub

Lock the door and fill the tub with warm water to the Jacuzzi level (above the highest jet)

The warm water will be therapeutic and will help ease the stiffness in your joints

While sitting in the tub you can begin doing alternate knee lifts and holding your knees for five seconds and then lowering them gently down until your feet are flat

Alternate your knee lifts for ten repetitions and two sets

Once you have completed your exercise relax and remember to drain the water before exiting the tub.

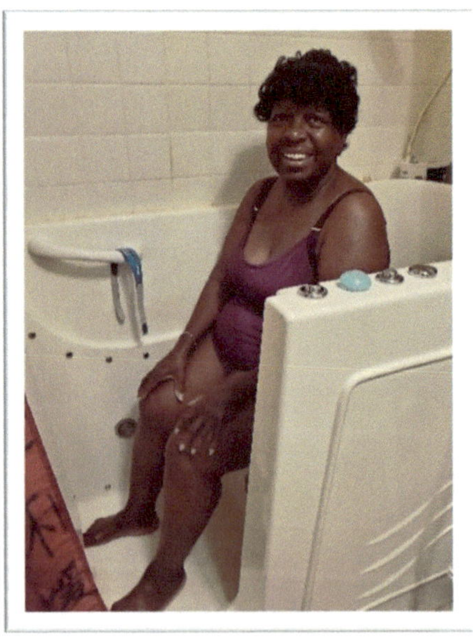
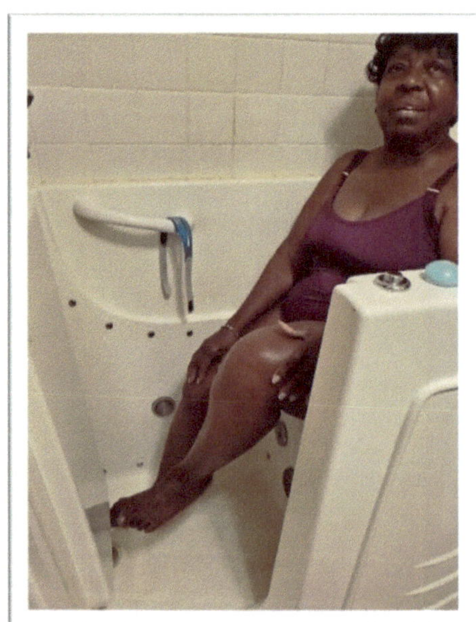

Section Four

Lying down

Exercises Part 2

Section 4-Pt.2-Lying down knee raise exercise

Directions

This exercise is for the lower body

Lay down on your bed and get comfortable

Raise your right knee as illustrated in the picture

Keep your foot flat and hold for ten seconds

Relax and lower your knee until your leg is in the starting position

Repeat exercise this exercise for ten repetitions

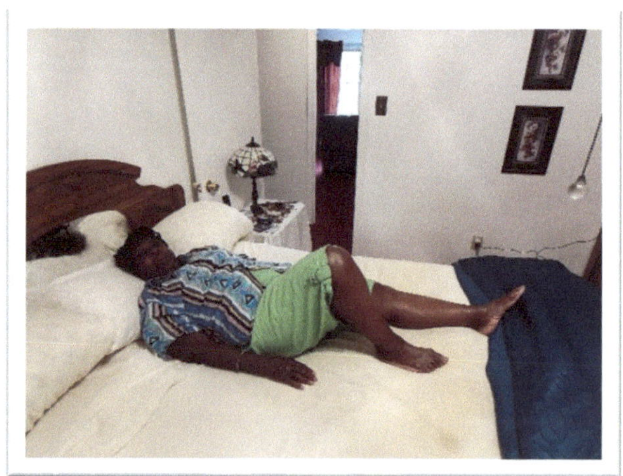

Lying down knee raise exercise

Directions

This exercise is for the lower body

Lay down on your bed and get comfortable

Raise your left knee as illustrated in the picture

Keep your foot flat and hold for ten seconds

Relax and lower your knee until your leg is in the starting position

Repeat exercise this exercise for ten repetitions

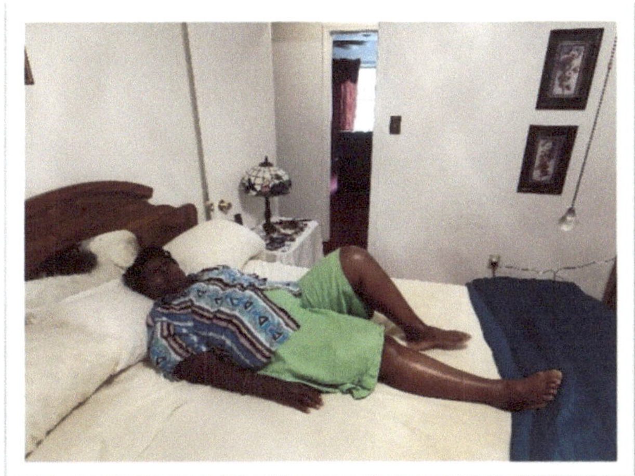

Left knee raise exercise

Alternate knee lying down exercise

Directions

This exercise is for the lower body

Lay down on your bed and get comfortable

Raise your right knee as illustrated in the picture

Keep your foot flat and hold for ten seconds

Relax and lower your knee until your leg is in the starting position

Alternate and raise your left knee and hold for ten seconds

Repeat exercise this exercise for ten repetitions and two sets

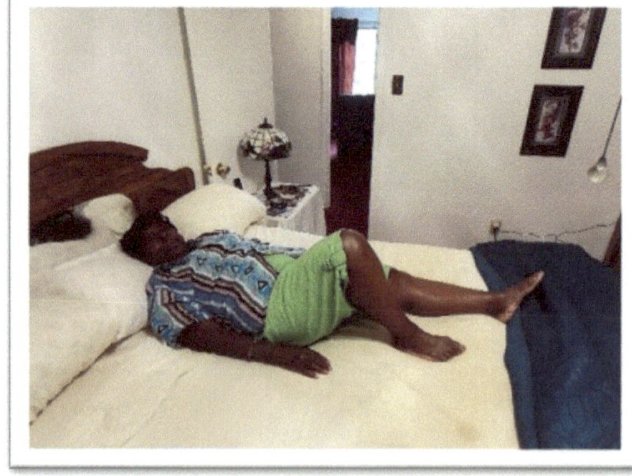
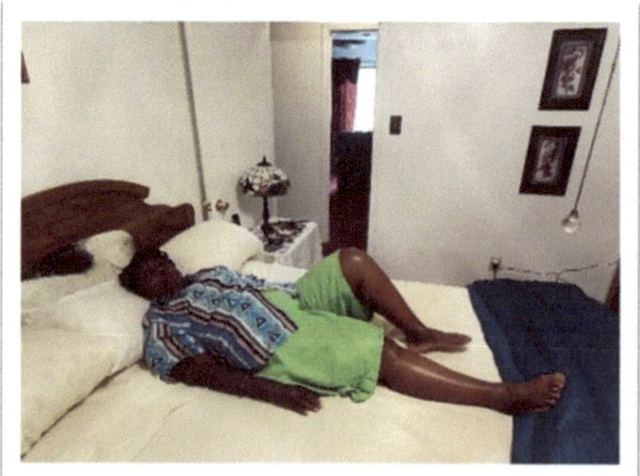

Section Five

Sitting

Exercises

Lifting Left Arm sitting exercise

Sit in a comfortable chair with your back straight and hands resting on your knees

Make sure both feet are flat on the ground

Take a moment and relax in the correct sitting position

Raise your left arm out to your side above your shoulder without straining yourself and hold for five seconds

Return to the starting position and wait five seconds and repeat this exercise.

Repeat this exercise for ten repetitions and two sets.

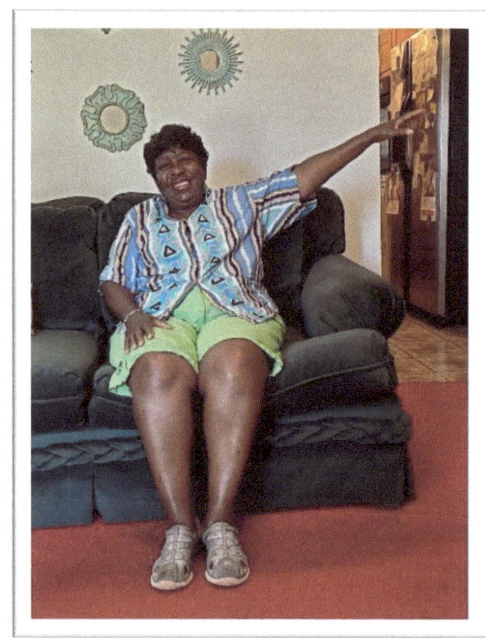

Lifting Right Arm sitting exercise

Sit in a comfortable chair with your back straight and hands resting on your knees

Make sure both feet are flat on the ground

Take a moment and relax in the correct sitting position

Raise your left arm out to your side above your shoulder without straining yourself and hold for five seconds

Return to the starting position and wait five seconds and repeat this exercise.

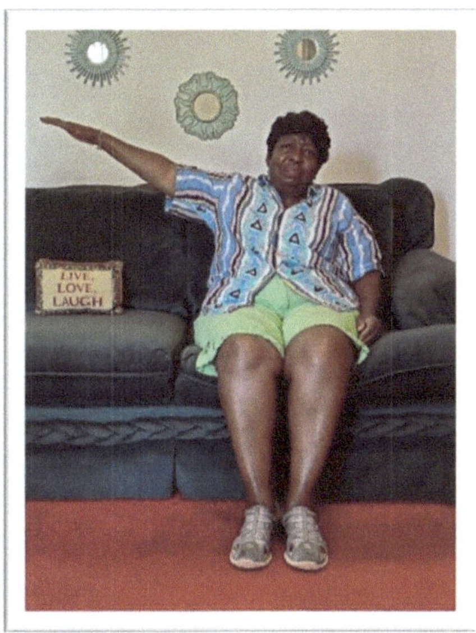

Sitting arm raise exercise

Alternate Arm lifting sitting exercise

Sit in a comfortable chair with your back straight and hands resting on your knees

Make sure both feet are flat on the ground

Take a moment and relax in the correct sitting position

Raise your left arm out to your side above your shoulder without straining yourself and hold for five seconds

Return to the starting position and wait five seconds and repeat this exercise

Alternate raising your right arm above your shoulder and hold for five seconds

Repeat each side for ten repetition and 2 sets.

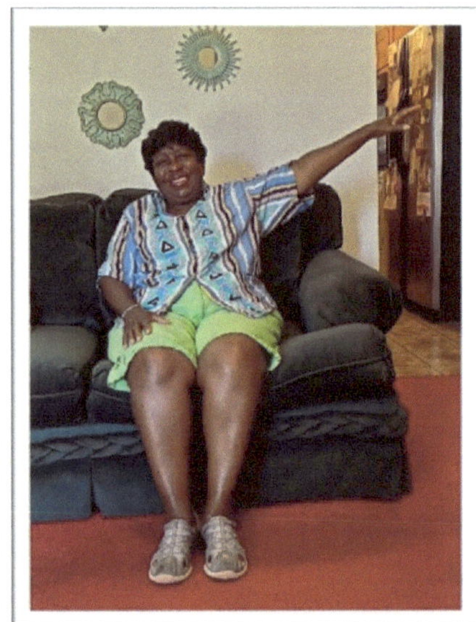 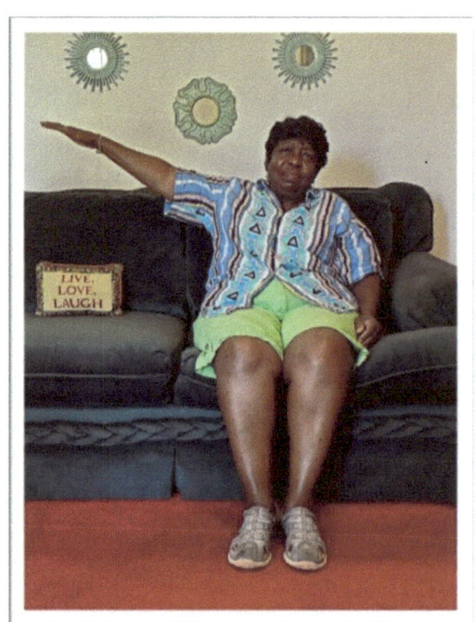

Siting alternate arm raising exercise

Chair upper body exercise
Lifting right arm to the front exercise

Directions

Sit in the chair with your bottom seated firmly

Take a moment to relax and get focus

Start with both hands resting upon your knees

Raise your right hand to the front until it is parallel with your shoulder or a little bit higher

Making sure you do not strain yourself

Hold this position for ten seconds and then lower your hand back to the starting position

Repeat this exercise for ten repetitions and two sets

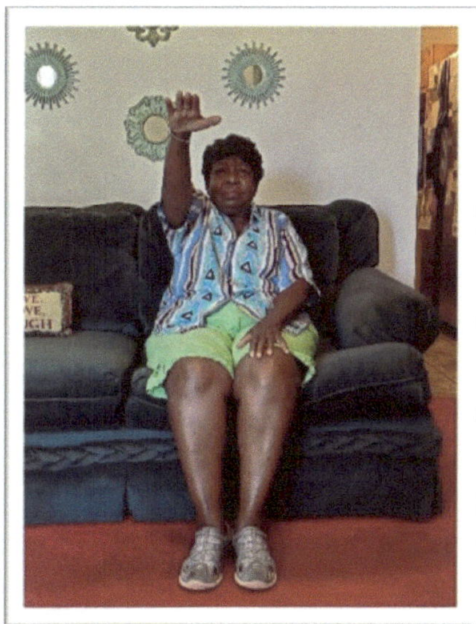

Chair upper body exercise
Lifting left arm to the front exercise

Directions

Sit in the chair with your bottom seated firmly

Take a moment to relax and get focus

Start with both hands resting upon your knees

Raise your left hand to the front until it is parallel with your shoulder or a little bit higher

Making sure you do not strain yourself

Hold this position for ten seconds and then lower your hand back to the starting position

Repeat this exercise for ten repetitions and two sets

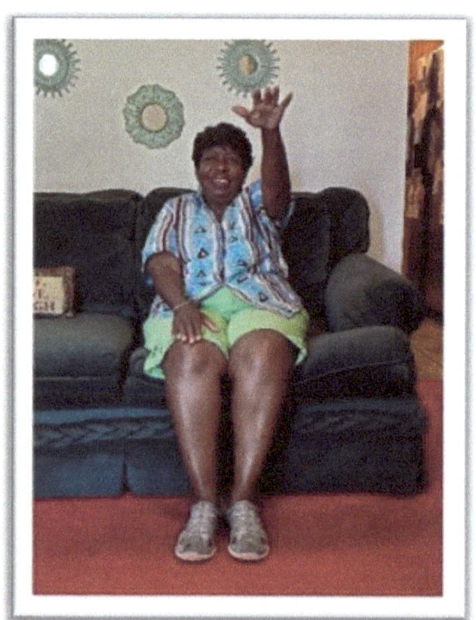

Chair upper body exercise
Alternate Lifting arm to the front exercise

Directions

Sit in the chair with your bottom seated firmly

Take a moment to relax and get focus

Start with both hands resting upon your knees

Raise your left hand to the front until it is parallel with your shoulder or a little bit higher

Making sure you do not strain yourself

Hold this position for ten seconds and then lower your hand back to the starting position

Alternate and raise your right hand and hold for ten seconds

Repeat this exercise for ten repetitions and two sets.

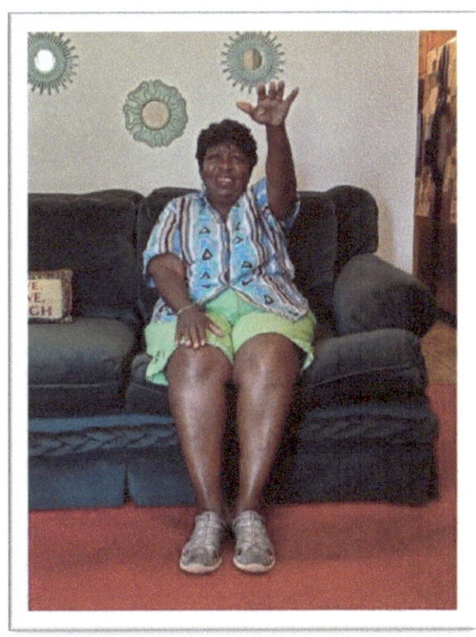
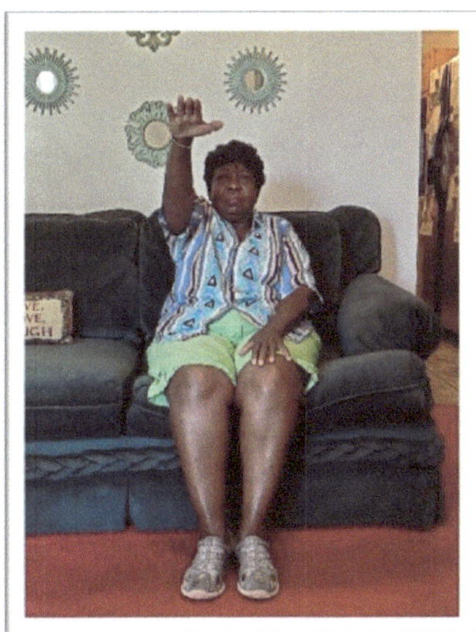

Section Six

Standing

Exercises

Section 6- Standing exercises

<u>Disclaimer As Mature Adults these exercises may be a little bit more difficult, so take your time.</u>

Directions

Stand with your back to the wall, and your feet flat and arms at your side facing forward

Let your hips touch the wall

As you gently lean back on the wall gradually raise your head as seen in the example picture

Keep facing the front as you stand relax keeping your back straight

Gradually turn your head to the right without straining and hold for ten seconds while standing from the wall keeping your posture straight

Return to the starting position and repeat this exercise ten times

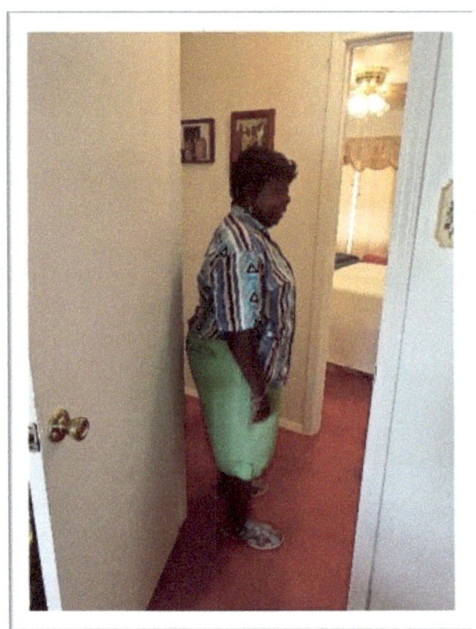 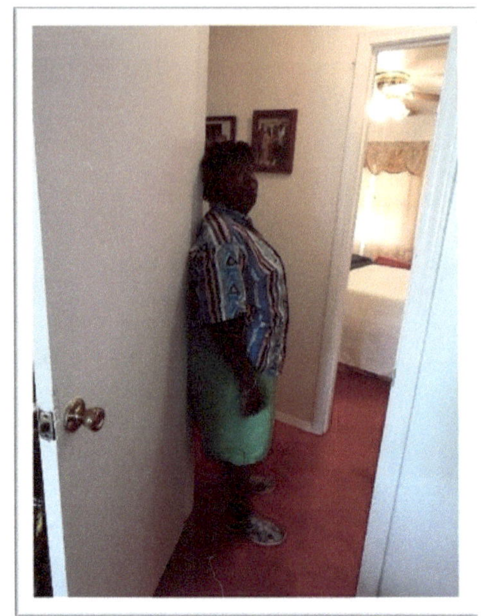

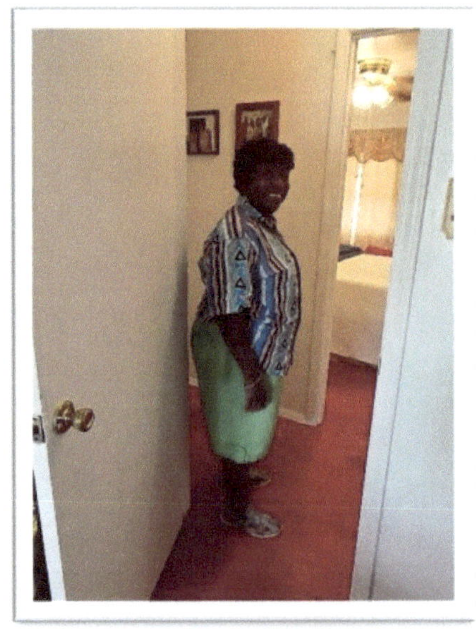 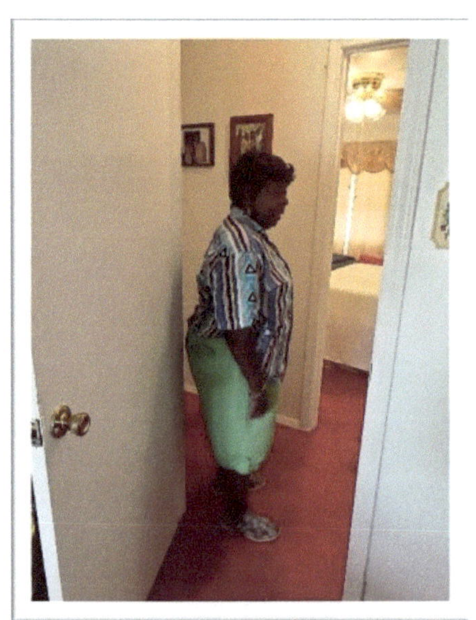

Section Seven

Pool

Exercises

Section 7- Pool Exercises

Water Aerobics
Note: You do not need to know how to swim to do water aerobics.

Directions

Shower before entering the pool

If available make sure you use the handrail and take your time entering the pool

Never try to carry anything in your hand while entering the pool

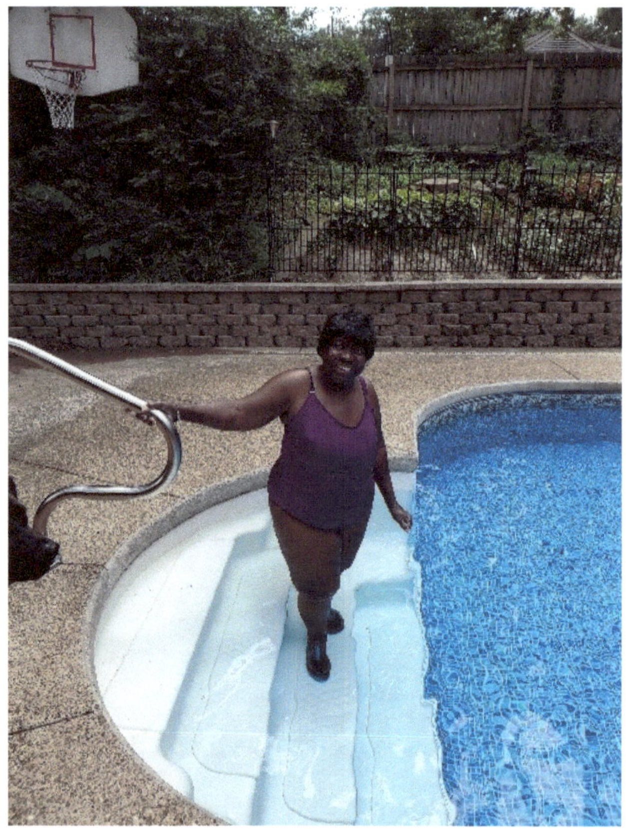

Water Aerobics Exercises

Jumping Jacks

Remember when you were young in school and the gym teacher made you do jumping jacks?
I am 76 years old and I enjoy doing jumping jacks in the pool, because the water keeps me feeling light and it is not such a jolt on my knees and joints.

Directions
Stand with your feel flat on the floor of the pool with arms at your side, and jump raising your hands up out of the water and standing out your feet keeping your balance.

Then return to starting position and repeat ten repetitions and two sets

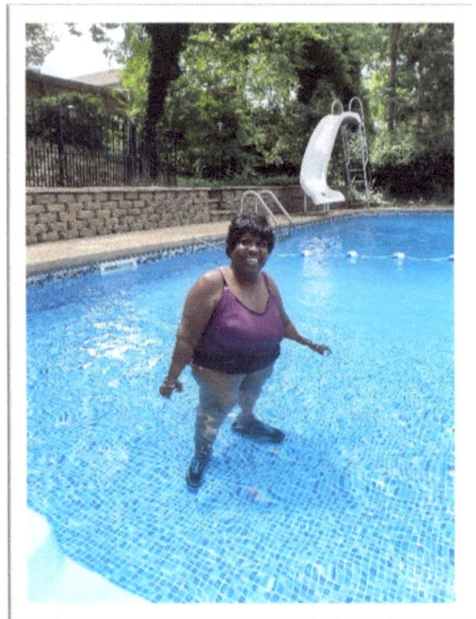

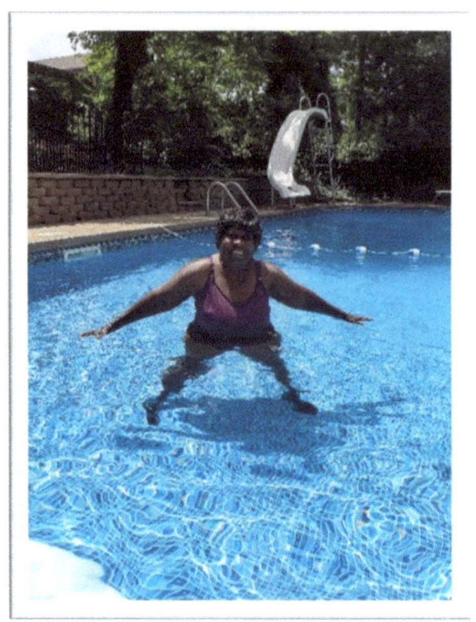

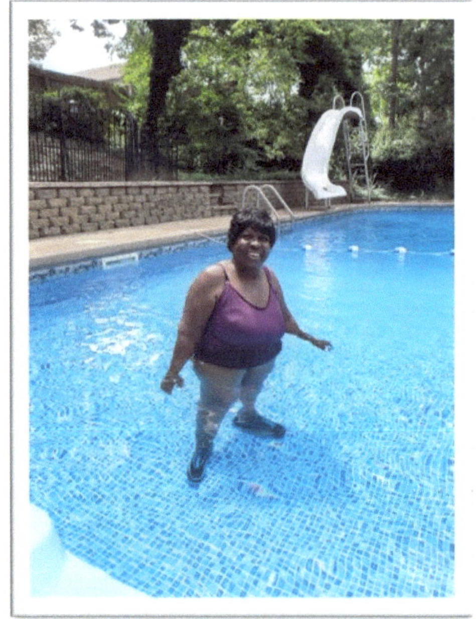

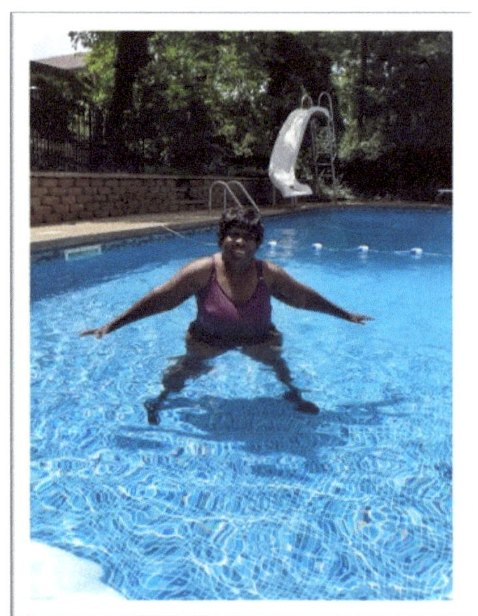

**Water jumping jacks
Pool Aerobics Exercises**

The Twist

Directions

This is an amazingly simple exercise that will help you stretch out your muscles and relax your joints

While standing in the pool with your feet flat hold your hands out to your sides keeping your hands in the water and then twist your body to the left and then to the right gently

If you are doing this exercise correctly you will see small circles forming in the water as you twist your body to the left and then the right

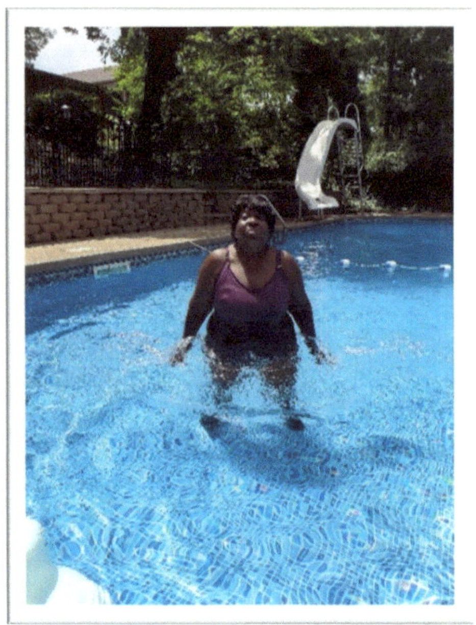
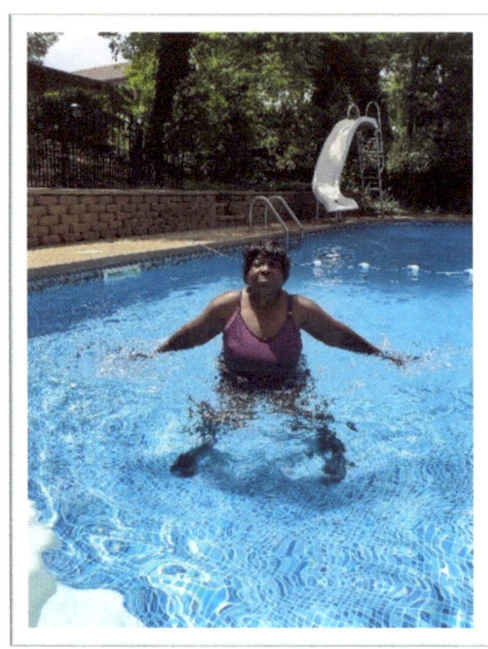

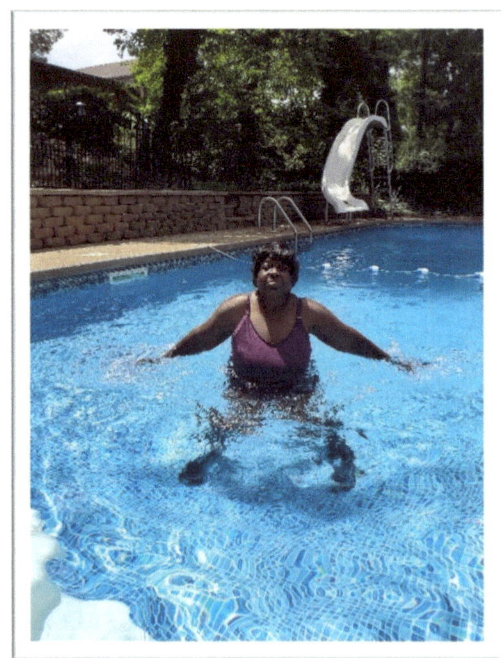
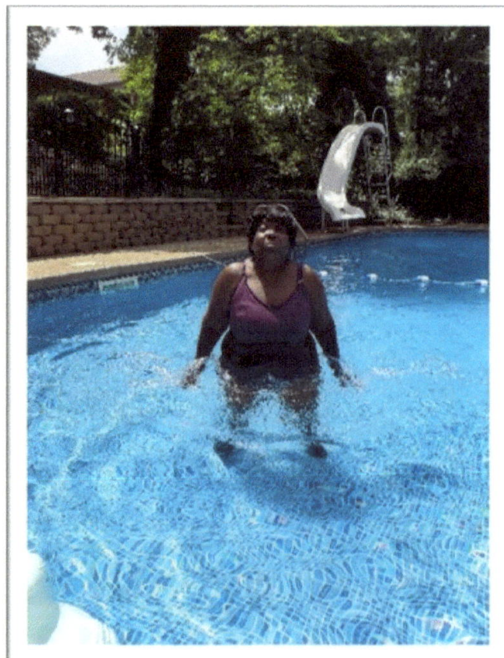

Water twist exercise

Section Eight

Standing from a Sitting position

Exercises

Section 8- Standing from a sitting position

Note: As mature adults the older we get the more difficult it is to stand from a sitting position so these exercises will strengthen your legs, back and joints so it will be easier for you to stand without struggling.

Sit with your back straight and feet planted firmly on the ground and hands flat on your knees

Lean forward with both hands going forward together and keeping your eyes to the front of you

Gradually use your legs and stand up keeping your knees relax but firm and straighten out your back

Continue this process until your standing fully and then you can lower your hands and move about freely

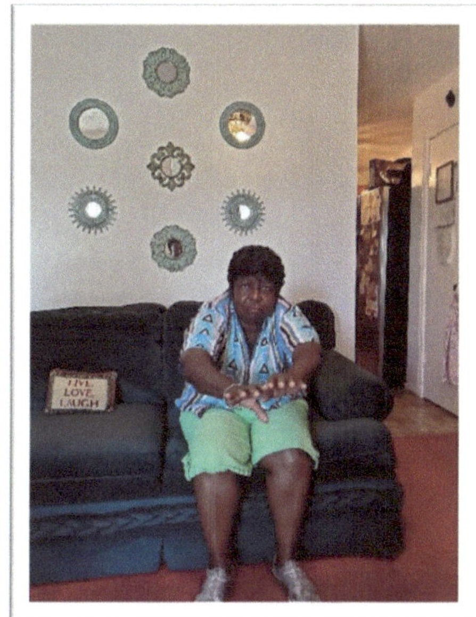

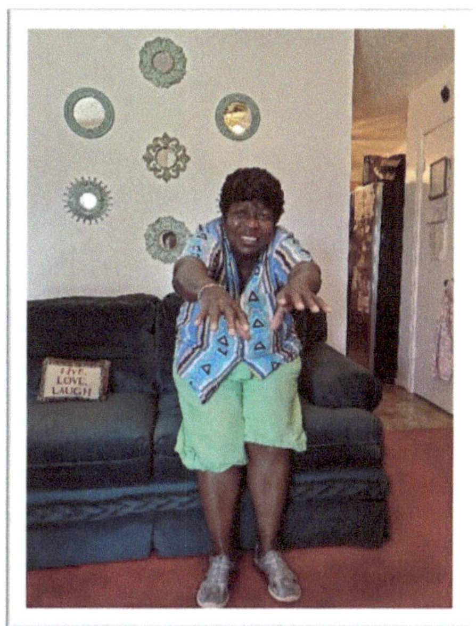

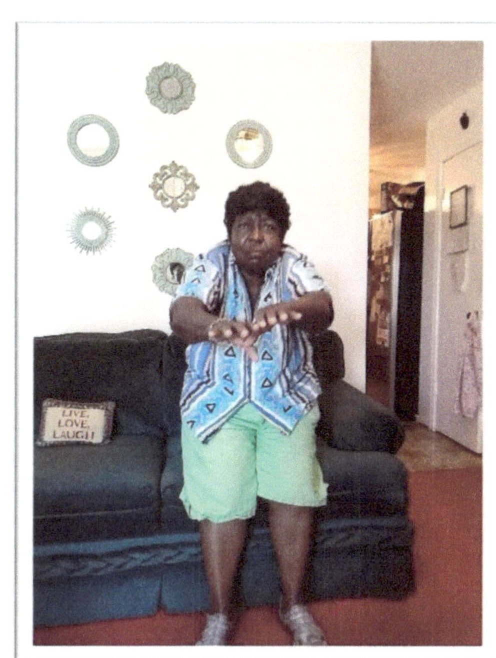

Standing from the sitting position

Pool

Exercise

Equipment

Government Regulated Equipment for indoor heated pools.

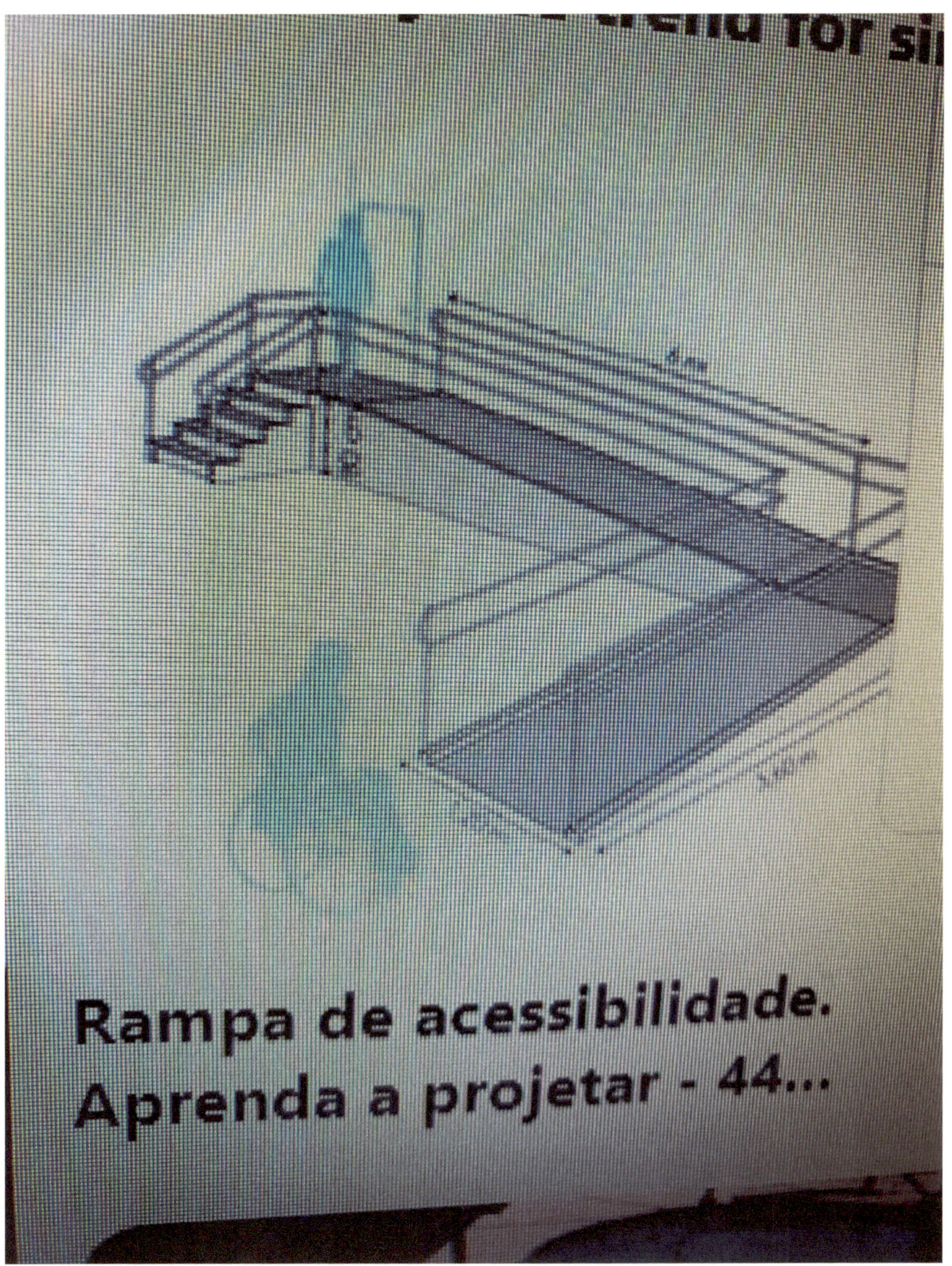
Rampa de acessibilidade.
Aprenda a projetar - 44...

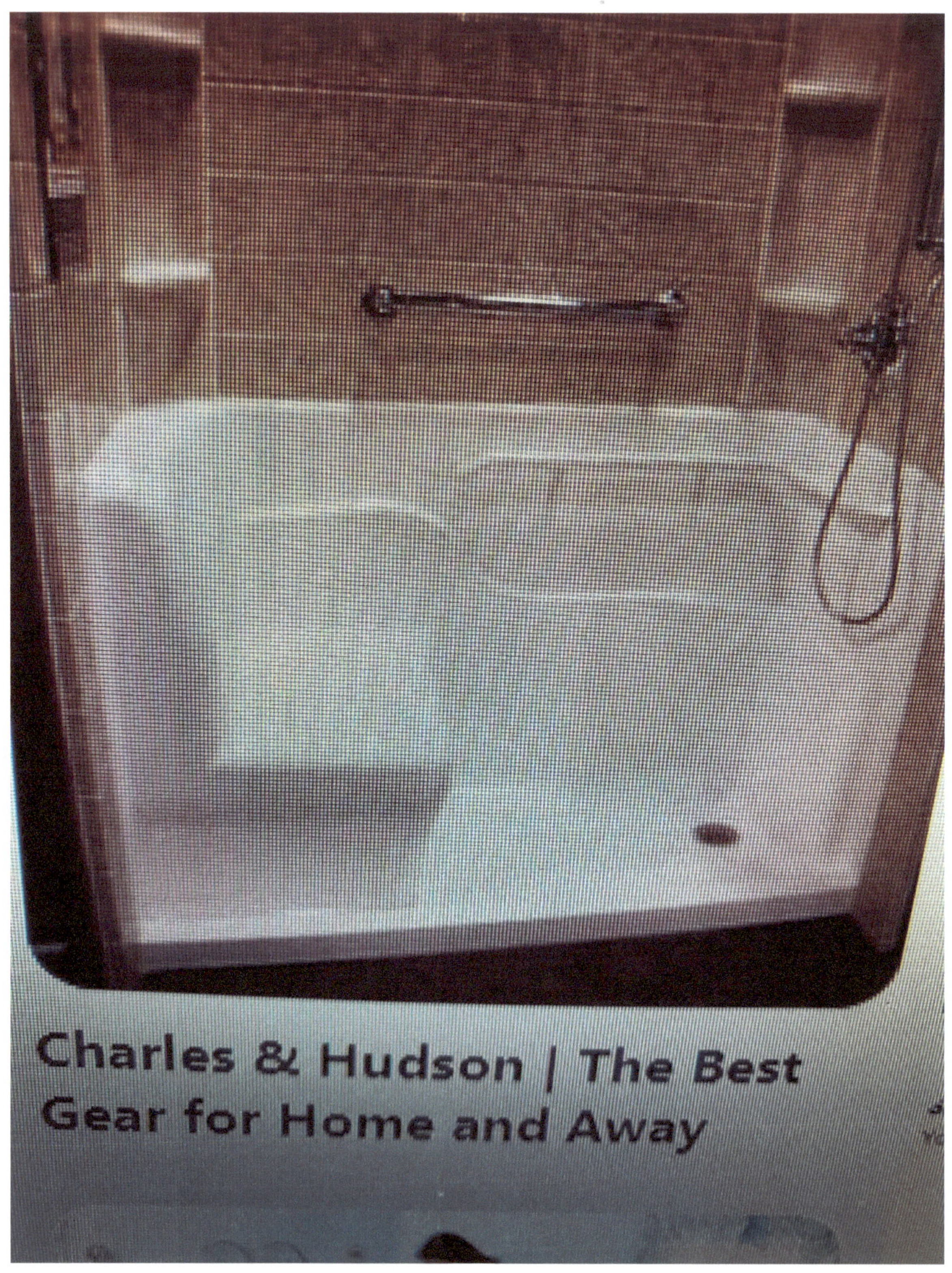
Charles & Hudson | The Best
Gear for Home and Away

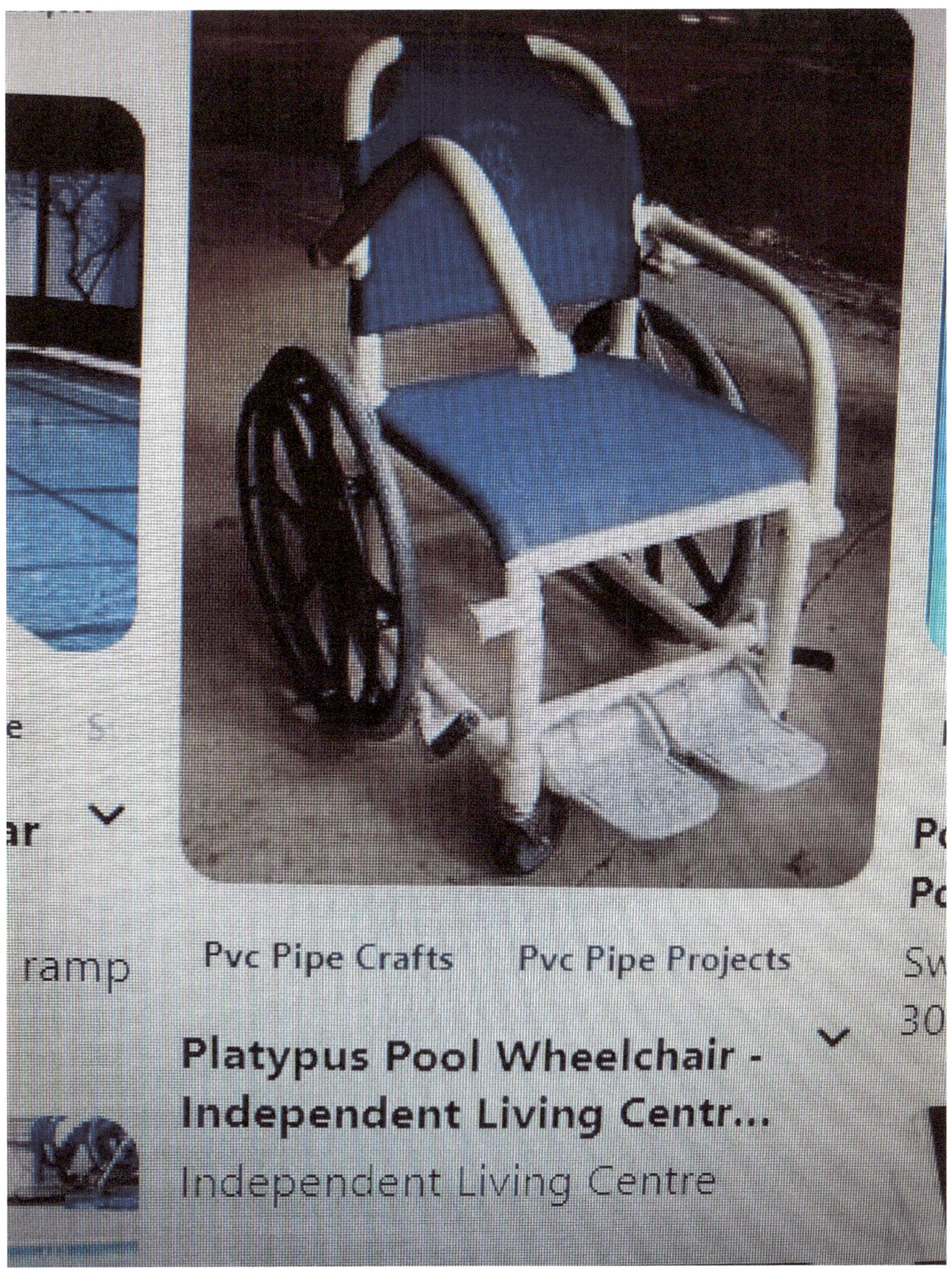
Pvc Pipe Crafts   Pvc Pipe Projects

Platypus Pool Wheelchair -
Independent Living Centr...
Independent Living Centre